Ostomy

I0469490

By Sharon C Kelly, Registered Nurse

• Glossary of terms • Ostomy supplies • Caring for your ostomy & stoma • Caring for your skin • Preventing skin infections • Problems that can occur with an ostomy • Conclusion • Resources

Do you have an ostomy? Are you concerned with how to deal with the changes to your body? Do you have questions about supplies and the different kinds of pouching systems? This article will answer these questions and more. I am a Registered Nurse who has worked in home health care and dealt first hand with people who have had ostomy surgery.

There is no question that this surgery can affect your body image but remember, this surgery can be lifesaving. Whether you have had the surgery for cancer or some other reason, you can get better and return to a normal life doing normal activities. One way to think of your ostomy is that it is just another way for you to have a bowel movement or pee.

Learning how to care for your ostomy, using the supplies that are right for you and your lifestyle, will make you feel better about it. Everyone with a new ostomy must deal with it in their own time and in their own way. Even though you may feel self conscious about your pouch and think everyone can see it through your clothes, this is not true. You probably cannot tell by looking at someone if they have a pouch on under their clothing. You will not need to purchase special clothing either, but you will want to avoid tight waistbands right over the stoma. Right after your surgery, your stoma will be quite large, but it will gradually shrink and reach its final size in six to eight weeks.

DIGESTIVE SYSTEM

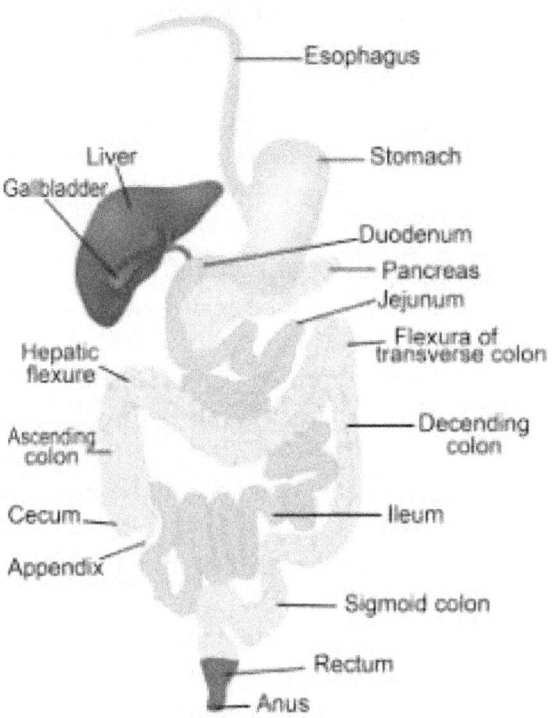

Esophagus

Liver

Gallbladder

Stomach

Duodenum

Pancreas

Jejunum

Flexura of transverse colon

Hepatic flexure

Ascending colon

Decending colon

Cecum

Ileum

Appendix

Sigmoid colon

Rectum

Anus

Glossary of terms

Many people get the word ostomy and stoma confused. These words have different meanings and, therefore, should not be used interchangeably.

Stoma: The actual end of the bowel or ureter that is protruding through the abdominal wall in order to let stool or urine exit the body. You won't be able to feel or control your urine or stool as it leaves your body through the stoma. When you look at the bowel stoma, you are actually seeing the lining of the intestine. It is warm, pink and moist and secretes small quantities of mucous.

Ostomy: The surgically formed fistula (opening) connecting a portion of the intestine or urinary tract to the exterior thru the abdominal wall.

Colostomy: Refers to the colon or large bowel.

Ileostomy: Refers to the ileum or small bowel.

Urostomy: Refers to a procedure that diverts the urine away from the bladder to the outside of the body. This is because the bladder is defective in some way, or has been removed.

Pouching system: A device worn over your stoma. This device acts as a reservoir for the urine or stool that empties out of the stoma. A system can have one or two pieces. In a one piece pouch, the pouch and skin barrier are attached together. In a two- piece system there is a skin barrier and a separate attachable pouch.

Skin barrier wafer: A solid square or round piece of adhesive material that is used to protect your skin from urine or stool.

WOCN: Wound, Ostomy, Continence Nurse – A nurse with specialized training in caring for people who have wounds, stomas, and/or bladder and bowel problems.

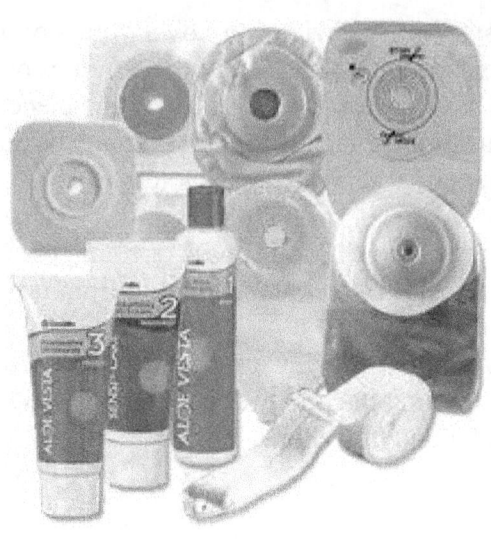

Ostomy Supplies

It is a good idea to reorder supplies several weeks before you expect them to run out in order to allow time for delivery. However, do not stockpile supplies because they do have a shelf life and also are affected by temperature changes.

Let's start with pouches for a colostomy. Pouches come in many styles and sizes. They are lightweight and lie flat against your body. You might need to try several different styles until you find the one that is right for you. Your WOC nurse can help you choose the one that is best for you. Pouches are made of disposable materials. Some are designed to be worn once and then disposed of. However, all pouches do the same job. They collect stool or urine. They contain the odor and they protect the skin around the stoma. The pouching system sticks to the skin around the stoma. Some are open at the bottom for easy emptying. You do not have to remove this type of pouch to empty it. It can remain in place for several days. Others are closed and are removed and thrown away when filled. They have no opening and cannot be emptied.

There are a variety of closure methods for drainable pouches. For colostomy and ileostomy drainable pouches, a clamp is used to close the pouch. When using a clamp, be sure to wrap the end or tail piece around the clamp only one time. Make sure it cannot slip off. Some pouches close without using a clamp. The pouch is sealed by folding or rolling the opening usually 3 times in the same direction. Velcro tabs secure the opening.

All **urostomy pouches** are drainable and have a valve that prevents urine from backing up around the stoma.
Pouches can be small or large. The size depends on how much stool or urine your body produces and your personal preference. Mini pouches are also available but have to be emptied or changed more often. These would be great to wear during intimate times.

Ostomy belts that attach to your pouch and lie level with the pouching system can be worn for extra support.

There are also **pouch covers** that come in a variety of prints. They hide the contents of the pouch and are soft against the skin.

Skin sealants also known as barrier film does not have to be used. They come in the form of sprays, wipes and gels and they put a plastic like coating on the skin. If you have skin that tears very easily, have trouble with leakage or are using a skin barrier powder, a skin sealant might help you. If you have dry or oily skin your pouching system may stick better with a skin sealant. Most skin sealants contain alcohol and if your skin has an open area the sealant will cause stinging, so make sure you get a non-sting sealant. Be sure you let the skin sealant dry completely before you apply the pouching system.

Adhesive remover is a product you can use if you need it. However, if you can remove your pouching system gently with water it is best not to use it. You do not want to use too many products on your skin. If your skin tears easily do not use adhesive remover. Some people will use adhesive remover to prevent the buildup of sticky residue on their skin. Because adhesive remover contains alcohol and feels oily, always wash well with mild soap and water to remove the oily coating on your skin. Then rinse the skin well with water and dry completely.

Ostomy skin barrier paste is used as a caulking to fill in gaps and creases. If your skin surface is wrinkly, the paste will help to even it out around the stoma. When your skin surface is even, you will get a better seal with the pouching system and therefore prevent leakage. You do not need to use paste if the skin around your stoma is smooth and you are getting a good fit with no leakage. To use the paste, apply it around the opening that you cut in the skin barrier. Use only a small bead of the paste and let it sit for one minute. This will give the alcohol in the paste a chance to evaporate. When trying to remove the paste from your skin, let it dry a little first. It is ok if a little bit of paste is left on your skin.

Ostomy skin barrier powder is used to dry a raw, weepy area on the skin. You only need to use powder if you are having a problem with your skin. If you do use powder, only use a light dusting. You can put a skin sealant over the powder before putting on your pouching system to help seal it better.

Ostomy adhesives are used to increase the stickiness between the pouching system and the skin. They are not used very often. If you use one, only a light, even coating should be used. Make sure the adhesive dries completely before putting on the pouching system. This is to help decrease the chance of chemicals in the adhesive from hurting your skin. It might take 3 to 5 minutes to dry. It is important to follow the manufacturer's directions completely.

Skin barrier wafers are either standard wear or extended wear. In general, a standard wear barrier is used when the stool is semi-formed or formed. An extended wear barrier does not break down like a standard wear barrier, when it comes in contact with loose to liquid drainage.

Caring for your Ostomy & Stoma

Using the right type of pouching system for your ostomy and putting it on correctly will determine how long you can wear it between changes. In addition to the type and proper fit, there are several other factors that can influence how long a pouch will stay sealed. These include weather, skin peculiarities, scars, weight changes, diet, activity, body contours near the stoma and the nature of your stool. Perspiration during summer months and warm humid climates may shorten the number of days you can wear your pouching system. Moist, oily skin may also reduce adhesion time. Many pouching systems are made to be worn for three to seven days. There are some however, that need to be changed every day. You can choose the type that is right for you.

The best time to change your pouching system is an individual matter. You want to have a time set aside when your stoma is not active and putting out a lot of drainage. This could be before eating or drinking in the morning or at the end of the day at least two hours after your evening meal. Because the stoma has no muscle, urine or stool may drain from your stoma while showering or bathing.

Yes, you can get your pouching system wet! You can shower, bathe, swim, and hot tub. Just be sure you empty your pouch first. You can take a bath or shower with your pouch on or off. Water will not enter the ostomy opening. In fact exposure to air and using soap and water will not do any harm to the stoma. However, only use a gentle spray of water on your stoma when showering.

As I said, your pouching system is waterproof, but you may feel more secure if you wear an ostomy belt or use waterproof tape to secure the edges of your skin barrier. You can use paper tape and wipe the tape with a skin sealant to make it more waterproof. This would be gentler on your skin. Gas filters do not work if they get wet, so protect them with waterproof tape. After bathing, you can use a towel or hairdryer on the coolest setting to dry the tape and pouching system in order to prevent skin irritation from wetness. You want to take your time when changing your pouching system. You do not want to rip the pouch off and consequently injure your skin. Loosen and lift the edges of the pouching system with one hand and push down on the skin near the skin barrier with the other hand. You may find it helpful to start at the top and work down. That way you can see what you are doing. Warm water works fine for some people in removing their pouching system. Other people use an adhesive remover. If you use an adhesive remover, be sure to wash your skin afterwards with soap and water and dry thoroughly. After you have removed your pouching system, empty the pouch in the toilet and then put pouch etc. in a plastic bag and then into the garbage. If you are using a reusable pouch follow the manufacturer's instructions for cleaning the pouch.

For cleaning around the stoma all you really need is warm water and a washcloth. It is not necessary to use soap but if you prefer too, make sure it is a mild soap with no perfumes, oils or deodorants in it. Perfumes etc. can sometimes cause skin problems and can also keep your skin barrier from sticking. Be sure to rinse your skin very well after using any kind of soap. If you are using paste, it might be easier to remove the paste before wetting your skin. A little bit of paste left on your skin will not hurt anything. Be gentle with your stoma. There are no nerve endings in the stoma, so you won't feel anything if you rub too hard. There are blood vessels in the stoma tissue, so you could see a small amount of blood on your washcloth after washing. Do not use any type of wipes (baby or otherwise) if they contain lanolin or other oils. Also, do not use powders or creams unless recommended by your doctor or WOC nurse.

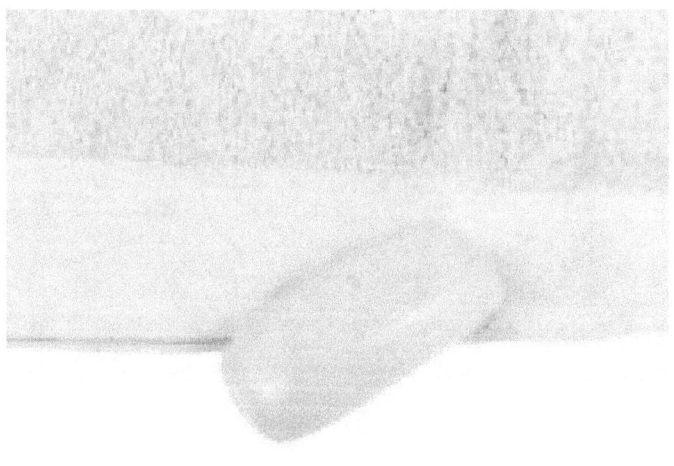

Caring for your skin

The best skin protection is a well-fitted and comfortable pouching system. The opening of your skin barrier should be no more than 1/8 inch away from the edge of your stoma. Measure your stoma once a week for the first six to eight weeks after your ostomy surgery. Your stoma will shrink while it is healing, therefore you need to measure it often during that time in order to make sure the opening in the skin barrier is not to large. Always re-measure your stoma if any skin irritation develops between your stoma and skin barrier wafer. Check your skin each time you change your pouching system. Use a mirror to check the skin under your stoma. Look for places where stool or urine may have leaked under the skin barrier and onto your skin. These areas may need some paste or skin barrier strips. This would be a good time to switch to an extended wear skin barrier if your stoma drains urine or loose stool.

It is recommended to change your pouch if itching or burning of your skin occurs. This may indicate a skin rash, or skin infection. Watch for any sensitivities and allergies to adhesives, skin barriers, tape or pouch material. These sensitivities can develop at any time, even weeks or months after the use of a product. You might try a pouch cover if you have skin irritation caused by pouch material.

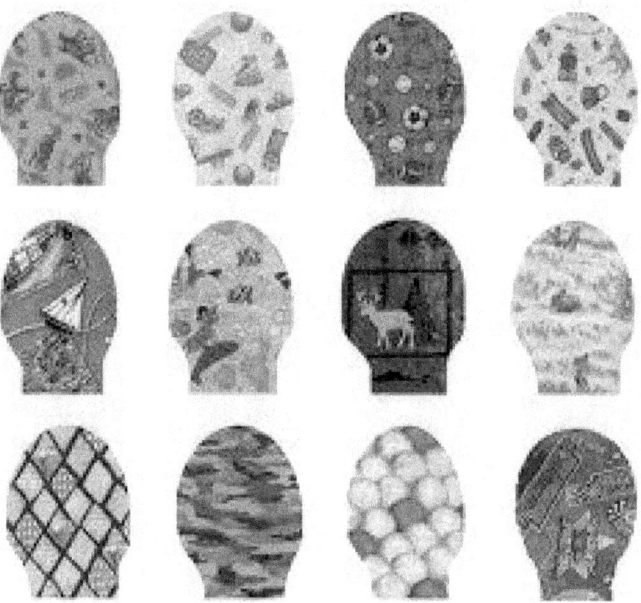

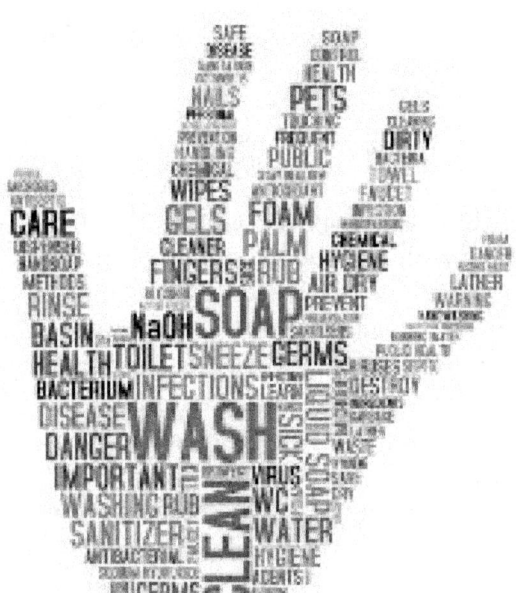

Preventing skin infections

The stoma is your bowel. It is protected by mucus so stool and urine won't hurt it. A stoma rarely becomes infected. The skin around the stoma is what you need to be careful of. Redness around the edges of the stoma while it is healing is normal If redness extends beyond 1/2 inch around the incision and you have pain or tenderness, discharge from the area, itchiness and redness, you may have an infection. If you think you have an infection, call your doctor or WOC nurse. A correct fitting pouching system is the best way to prevent an infection of your skin. Be sure to change your pouching system at the first sign of leakage. Do not try to patch the pouching system with tape or paste. Empty your pouch before it becomes half full and release gas before your pouch gets too full. You don't want to put stress on the bag and risk it leaking. If you are bothered by a lot of gas, you might want to try a pouch that has a vent or filter in it. The gas will lesson after your bowel has had time to heal from the surgery and you are able to tolerate a regular diet. You might want to keep a food diary in order to see what foods you are not tolerating well.

Problems that can occur with an ostomy

Call you doctor or WOC nurse for any of the following problems:

- The most common problem after a colostomy surgery is the development of a hernia around the stoma site. This can usually be prevented by not lifting heavy objects right after surgery.

- Diarrhea if it lasts more than two days. It usually comes on suddenly and can be accompanied by abdominal cramping. Dehydration can occur with diarrhea, so drink at least 8-10 glasses of fluid such as pedialyte or water.

- Blood in your pouch (over four tablespoons) and if you have more than a spot of blood coming from your stoma.

- Your stoma changes size or looks different. Your stoma should appear pink, red and moist. If your stoma becomes a dark purplish red color, this could mean there is not enough blood being supplied to the stoma. Also, the stoma should not protrude higher than the surrounding skin or sink below the skin surface.

- Your ileostomy or urostomy has no output for four to six hours. You could have an obstruction, especially if you have accompanying cramps or nausea

- Severe skin breakdown that does not improve.

- Severe cramping lasting more than two or three hours.

- Unusual odor lasting more than a week.

- Severe injury to the stoma.

- Watery discharge lasting more than five or six hours.

- Narrowing of the stoma.

- Suddenly having to change your pouching system more often than usual.

Conclusion

I hope this article has helped you to understand your ostomy and stoma a little bit better. Learning to live with an ostomy may seem like an overwhelming problem at times but remember there is no reason why you cannot do after your ostomy, what you did before the ostomy. This is one of those life changing situations and it is normal to feel discouraged at times. You may want to talk to someone when you are feeling down. You will have to adapt to a new way of life, but you do not have to do it alone. There is lots of support out there for you. See resource list.

God Bless!

Resources

United Ostomy Associations of America, Inc. 1-800-826-0826

Wound, Ostomy and Continence Nurses - national office, 1-800-224-9626 or visit www.wocn.org

www.ostomyworld.com

www.cmostomysupply.com

www.stlmedical.com

About the author

Sharon Kelly is a Registered Nurse who is currently working with nursing students at a local Community College. She has done hospital nursing, home health & hospice nursing, and nursing education. She may be contacted at:

www.skillsfornurses.com

www.thehomecarer.com